CREATE YOUR OWN ANTI-INFLAMMATORY GROCERY LIST

A Focus On What You Can Eat. Not What You Can't

With tips on foods and ingredients from every grocery store section that are gluten free, dairy free, soy free and nightshade free. Including Brand Name Foods to look for.

By Paula C. Henderson

ISBN: 9798624627109

Amazon Authors Page:
www.amazon.com/author/paulachenderson

Table of Contents

We focus so much on what we can't eat that it really becomes difficult and sometimes depressing to try and come up with what we actually can eat.

Lets focus on all the many foods you can eat. The truth is the the majority of foods are gluten free, dairy free, soy free and nightshade free. We will only eliminate gluten, dairy, soy, and nightshades. I have included tips for those of you also avoiding grains like oats, corn and rice.

Take this booklet to the grocery store with you (you will only need to do this once) and create your master list of foods you already like or would like to try that are gluten free, dairy free, soy free and nightshade free. From here you can create meal plans and menu's.

Walk each aisle and department of your favorite grocery store. As you walk through each department of your grocery store write down all of the products that are gluten free, dairy free, soy free and nightshade free that you already like or that you would like to try.

Compiling this list of WHAT YOU CAN EAT will go a long way to easing your anxieties and you will find yourself referring to it weekly when making your grocery list.

Not all foods are marked Gluten Free, Dairy Free, Soy Free and/or Nightshade Free. The following foods are naturally okay to eat and will most likely not have any statement printed on the food product packaging:

Naturally Gluten Free, Dairy Free, Soy Free and Nightshade Free:

- All meats and seafoods. All. Without seasonings. Fresh, frozen, canned.
- All fruit except goji berries. All. Fresh, frozen, canned.
- All vegetables except: soybean products, eggplant, tomatoes, tomatillos, peppers, white potatoes. Fresh, frozen, canned.

Also Avoid: soy sauce, tofu, soybeans, edamame, paprika, red pepper, anything with wheat flour or cows milk.

I have two booklets for those who need more assistance on choosing foods. Each contain a comprehensive list of thousands of products from every aisle of the grocery store that meet the requirement to assist you in making your own list. I read the ingredients list of every item before deciding to put it on the list. I included brand named packaged products as well as those food items in the meat/seafood and produce aisle that do not have packaging.

1. A Comprehensive Gluten & Dairy Free Grocery List: Over 1000 Food Items From Every Dept: ISBN: 1098618084
2. A Comprehensive Gluten & Dairy Free, Soy Free and Nightshade Free Grocery List: ISBN: 9798625037518

REFRIGERATED

Some dairy-free products include soymilk and if you are avoiding soy you will want to avoid those. ***You will find that the same brand will have some varieties with soy and others without soy. Be sure to glance at the ingredients list even within the same brand.*** Watch out for dips, hummus and prepared guacamole as sometimes it will have whey (dairy) or nightshades like jalapeno added.

Eggs________

DAIRY FREE BUTTER ALTERNATIVES:

DAIRY FREE MILK

DAIRY FREE YOGURT

....

....

....

BEVERAGES

All juices are okay with the exception of tomato juice
which is a nightshade. Tea is also okay.
Check the label in your refrigerated beverage section.
Avoid any ingredient like milk, soy, whey, tomato, *spices.

....

....

....

....

....

....

....

....

....

BEVERAGES

Water is best! Avoid dairy like whey and milk. Avoid nightshades like tomato and vague spices in the ingredients list like *spices. Avoid anything with soy. Most beverages in the Beverage Aisle are gluten free, soy free, dairy free and nightshade free such as most juices (not V8 or tomato), soda, lemonade, kool-aid and punch.

Avoid hot cocoa mixes and instead buy a Chocolate Dairy Free Milk and heat it up. Marshmallows are a clean food so you can add those too! Coffee and tea are also a clean approved food.

Avoid beer unless it states Gluten Free. Wine and Tequila are okay.

Hershey's Milk Chocolate Syrup (original) is clean! Yeah! Read the label if buying a different Hershey's variety like low fat, dark chocolate or others.

BAKING AISLE

FLOUR AND STARCHES

Avoid anything with the ingredient soy, soybean, wheat, and potato flour or potato starch. If you are also avoiding grains you will want to avoid oats, rice, and corn (cornmeal). These grains are naturally gluten free but some people are sensitive to them. Many brands are making a Gluten Free variety that you can try.

Here is a short list of gluten free nightshade free flours:

- Amaranth
- Almond
- Arrowroot
- Buckwheat
- Cassava
- Chickpea
- Corn starch
- Coconut
- Millet
- Oat
- Rice
- Sorghum
- Tapioca
- Teff

- Gluten free oat flour
- Gluten free corn meal

Starches are included above: Corn starch, tapioca and arrowroot. Many gluten free recipes call for Xanthan Gum and can be found in most grocery stores. Xanthan gum gives breads that sort of gluten elasticity texture.

Baking soda and Baking powder are gluten free.

FLOUR AND STARCHES

ALL SUGAR IS GLUTEN FREE, DAIRY FREE, NIGHTSHADE FREE AND SOY FREE.

- Agavi
- Brown Sugar
- Honey
- Powdered Sugar
- Stevia
- White Sugar

....

....

....

....

An example of why you should read your labels.
The first ingredient on the Jiffy Corn Muffin Mix is Wheat Flour.

Oil

When you see the oil labels VEGETABLE OIL please turn it around and read the ingredient list. Its pure soybean oil. Avoid this oil. Watch out for blends. Many blends have soybean oil. Just read the label. Otherwise, use the oil that you works best for you.

....

....

....

....

SEASONING AND SPICES

The following seasoning and spices are nightshades:

- Ashwagandha
- Cayenne Pepper
- Chili Pepper Flakes
- Chili Powder
- Chinese Five Spice Powder
- Crushed Red Pepper
- Garam Masala
- Paprika

Packets and Spice Blends that include a long list of ingredients (check them first if you wish) Many packets and blends also include gluten and some have dairy.

- Black pepper and White pepper are not nightshades.
- Cumin is not a nightshade.

Seasonings and Spices

....

....

....

....

....

....

....

....

....

....

....

FLAVORS AND EXTRACTS

All flavoring and extracts are okay so long as it does not include malt, whey, milk, or nightshades such as peppers. The most common are vanilla flavoring or vanilla extract, mint and almond extract, for example, which are all clean. Food colorings are also okay.

- Avoid dairy like condensed milk and evaporated milk, but canned coconut milk is fine.
- Cocoa Butter is okay, it is not dairy.
- Butterfat **is** a dairy so avoid that. Butterfat is an ingredient in most chocolate chips and in many icings.
- The original Hershey's Milk Chocolate Syrup is okay!
- Coconut flakes are okay!
- Marshmallows are okay!
- All nuts and seeds are okay.
- Canned pumpkin is also okay!
- Unsweetened Baking Cocoa is okay!
- Graham Crackers are a gluten.
- Most canned fruit pie filling is also clean and okay to buy. Check the label.
- Most pie crust are not gluten free, but there the Mi-Del Gluten Free Graham Style Pie Crust is okay.
- Goats Milk: Most people find goats milk bothers them like cow's milk while a few say it's a great alternative.

Not all icing, even within the same brand are treated alike. Watch out for whey, soy, milk, and butterfat and avoid those ingredients. I have a comprehensive list in my book: A Comprehensive Anti-Inflammatory Grocery List: Gluten Free, Dairy Free, Soy Free and Nightshade Free – Includes prepared brand name foods. One icing that is clean is Pillsbury Creamy Supreme Cream Cheese Frosting, which is not one you would expect, right? Is it healthy? No, but none of the ingredients are dairy. It does contain a small trace amount of soy lecithin and if you are very sensitive to soy you might want to avoid this product. However, most people can tolerate minute amounts on rare occasion and seeing as how this is a product one would not use regularly I include it in my list of approved foods. As with any food, if you find it bothers you just eliminate it from your diet.

MIXES

Cake mixes, pudding mixes, bread mixes and more.
Many of the pudding mixes are okay. Just check the label. The prepared puddings usually have milk so you will want to avoid those. All Jell-O mixes are okay as well as prepared jello.

BREAKFAST AISLE

This is a very highly processed food aisle but if you find your body is okay with that so long as it is dairy free, gluten free and soy free than here are some tips. Avoid wheat, whey, soy, milk, bleached flour. Try gluten free oats if you are bothered by regular oats. If you are still bothered you may have a sensitivity to grains (oats, rice and corn).

RICE AND DRIED BEANS

Rice and dried beans are naturally gluten free, dairy free, soy free and nightshade free. The exception would be edamame which are soybeans.

Many are avoiding legumes and grains. You only need do this if you are sensitive to these foods. For me, I was chronically constipated for 8 years. I avoided gluten and dairy for joint pain reasons and that helped the pain but I was still constipated. When I decided a year later to try avoiding all grains and legumes I was suddenly cured of my constipation. The opposite of what the doctors told me to do. Having said that, that will not be the case for everyone. I found after 4 months of zero grains and legumes I am now able to tolerate the occasional serving about once a month or so.

Avoid packets with seasoning like Knorr Sides, Zatarain's, Rice a Roni, Uncle Bens Ready Rice and Near East.

Look for packages labeled gluten free or brown rice pasta. If you are very sensitive to nightshades watch out for potato starch in the ingredients list. Avoid boxed potatoes and stuffing.

....

....

....

INTERNATIONAL FOODS

There are foods like Old El Paso Taco Shells that are made with just limed corn flour, palm oil and salt for those of you who can tolerate corn ingredients. As we stated earlier, corn is naturally gluten free. There is sometimes cross contamination during manufacturing and that is why those with very sensitive allergies avoid corn.

....

....

....

....

....

....

....

....

CONDIMENTS

- While peanuts are a clean food, most major brands include soybean oil in the making of their peanut butter. Look for a peanut or nut butter that does not use soybean oil. Most jelly, jams and preserves are okay to eat.
- Pickles and relish can sometimes have nightshades such as dehydrated red pepper, or *spices, but, it is fairly easy to find varieties that do not. Check the label.
- Mayo and Salad Dressings like Miracle Whip traditionally use soybean oil. But it is pretty easy these days to find one that avoids soybean oil. Start by looking for one labeled Avocado Oil or Olive Oil Mayo and check the label to be sure.
- If you can find a mustard without paprika. Stick with those limited to vinegar, water, mustard seed, salt and turmeric. Not paprika.
- Olives are okay with the exception of olives with pimento. The olive is okay, not the pimento which is a nightshade. Stick to black olive and Kalamata olives
- Lea & Perrins is a gluten free Worcestershire sauce **but** it has Chili pepper extract as the last ingredient so if you are super sensitive to nightshades than you should avoid this product or limit your usage.

CANNED FOODS

- Avoid 'seasoned' products, and some soups like cream of soups. Check your labels as some soups are fine. Surprisingly many have wheat and dairy that you would not expect.
- Your best choice is single product canned goods like green beans, carrots, peas.
- When choosing canned meats, again, avoid seasoned.
- Stick with items like plain canned tuna and chicken (but avoid those in soybean oil). Things like canned mushrooms and unseasoned canned artichokes, and bamboo shoots, hearts of palm and water chestnuts are okay.
- Remember that all fruits (except goji berries), meats and seafood's are clean. You just have to be sure, with packaged food, that there are not added ingredients you should be avoiding.

FREEZER

Stick with unseasoned products.

····································   ····································

····································   ····································

····································   ····································

····································   ····································

····································   ····································

····································   ····································

····································   ····································

MEAT AND SEAFOOD

All meats and seafood's, without added ingredients are clean and okay to eat.

····································   ····································

····································   ····································

····································   ····································

····································   ····································

····································   ····································

····································   ····································

····································   ····································

PRODUCE

All fruits (except goji berries) and all vegetables except nightshades are okay.
Nightshades: russet and Idaho potatoes, red potatoes, tomatoes, tomatillos, eggplant, all peppers like bell peppers and hot peppers. Sweet potatoes and yams are okay.

COOKIES AND CRACKERS

Most cookies and crackers are made from wheat but there are some rice crackers like Nabisco Thins Gluten Free Corn & Rice Crackers that are okay to consume.

CHIPS AND SNACKS

- Plain popcorn is naturally gluten free and okay to eat.
- Nuts, seeds and dried fruits are okay. Jerky can sometimes include soy sauce and nightshades so check your ingredients list.
- Unseasoned pork rinds/pork skins are okay.
- Some corn chips and corn tortilla chips are okay but you need to check the label.

CANDY AND GUM

- Things like Sweetarts and Gummies are generally okay; check the label. Most chocolate candy bars are not.
- Twizzlers and Good & Plenty Licorice actually has wheat flour. A place you would not expect to find it.
- Many gums and mints that are otherwise okay to eat have small amounts of soy lecithin. Check your labels.
- If you like those fruity freezer pops you're in luck. Most that I checked are okay. Just glance at the label first.
- Fruit flavored suckers and lollipops and jolly ranchers are generally okay.

BREADS AND TORTILLAS

Look for packages clearly marked Gluten Free. If you are especially sensitive to nightshades avoid those with potato starch and potato flour in the ingredients list.

BRANDS TO LOOK FOR

Many of your favorite traditional brands are now offering gluten and dairy free options so be sure to check them first. Here is a list of fairy new brands finding their way into your grocery store that focus many or all of their products on gluten and dairy free that you can also look for in the store.

BFree

– Web site: www.bfreefoods.com

Clean products that are gluten free, dairy free, soy free and nightshade free:

- Gluten Free White Loaf: Gluten free, dairy free, soy free and nightshade free.
- White Demi Baguettes

Not Clean Products:

- Brown Seeded Sandwich Loaf: includes potato flour
- Soft White Sandwich Loaf
- The BFree Sweet Potato & Cinnamon Dinner rolls however have nightshades which includes potato starch, potato flour and tomato powder.
- The main ingredient in their plain Dinner Rolls is potato starch; a nightshade.
- All of their tortillas include potato flour as a main ingredient. If you have eliminated nightshades you will want to avoid those.
- Plain and Multiseed Bagel: includes potato starch and potato fiber
- Pita Bread includes potato flour as a main ingredient.

Barilla

- www.barilla.com

Barilla offers gluten free, dairy free, soy free and nightshade free elbow macaroni, spaghetti, lasagna sheets, fettuccine, rotini, and penne. They use a combination of corn and rice flours. If you are avoiding grains you will want to avoid pasta of all kinds.

Not all Barilla products are gluten free. Their Gluten Free line is clearly marked on the front of the package.

Clean Products:

Almond Breeze Horchata is gluten free, dairy free, soy free and nightshade free. It does show rice flour as an ingredient for those of you avoiding grains.

Almond Milk: all the varieties are clean. Original, Chocolate, Vanilla, Unsweetened Vanilla, Unsweetened Chocolate, Hint of Honey Vanilla, Reduced Sugar Almond milk, and the Unsweetened Original.

I am so excited that Almond Breeze now offers an Unsweetened Chocolate Almond milk

Coconut and Cashew Milks: All clean.

I noticed on their web site they now have an Almond Breeze Almond Milk with Real Bananas. Find with the other Almond Milk in the refrigerated section of your grocery store.

Almondmilk Creamer: All clean.

Almondmilk Yogurt Alternative:

Clean:

- Original: clean
- Vanilla: clean
- +Coconut flavored diced almonds & dark chocolate chips: clean
- +Honey Roasted Almonds & Granola: clean (note this does include oats and rice products.
- +Chocolate Flavored Almonds & Dark Chocolate: clean
- +Blueberry Flavored Almonds & Oat Cluster: Clean (oats and rice warning)
- +Toasted Almonds

Not Clean:
- +Salted Caramel Flavored Almonds and Pretzels: includes gluten from the wheat flour in making the pretzels and the ingredient malt.

Bob's Red Mill has a gluten free line of products.

Clean Products (ie: gluten free, dairy free, soy free, nightshade free)
- All of the Gluten Free Granola
- Oat Bars are also clean; even the chocolate
- Gluten Free flours: coconut, hazelnut, almond, cassava
- Chia Seeds
- Muesli: all three varieties
- Bob's Red Mill Grain Free Paleo Pancake & Waffle Mix: clean

Not Clean:

- Gluten Free Pancake Mix has potato starch. A nightshade.
- Gluten Free Brownie Mix has potato starch.
- Gluten Free Vanilla Yellow Cake Mix has potato starch.
- Gluten Free Pie Crust has potato starch.
- Gluten Free Muffin Mix has potato starch.
- Gluten Free Pizza Crust Mix has potato starch.

Bob's Red Mill will clearly state on the front of the package if the product is Gluten Free.

Bragg

- www.bragg.com

Bragg Organic Raw Unfiltered Apple Cider Vinegar "with the mother" is what I use for my Fatigue Fighting Tea. Hot, cold or room temp. I make a pitcher each week so that I have at least 8 ounces a day ready to drink. I have tried regular apple cider vinegar and I have tried the apple cider vinegar supplements. They do not work for fighting the chronic fatigue cause by RA and hypothyroidism. I make a pitcher of decaf tea and add the vinegar and honey to taste in a pitcher. Enough for the week. 3 parts vinegar to 1 part vinegar and then enough Raw Honey (not regular honey) to taste so I can actually drink it.

- Avoid the Liquid Aminos if you are avoiding soy. While it is gluten free it contains soy sauce.
- Bragg Organic Sprinkle Seasoning has nightshades.
- Bragg Organic Vinaigrette includes Liquid Aminos in the ingredients list. Their Liquid Aminos includes soy sauce. It is otherwise gluten and dairy free as well as nightshade free.
- Bragg Ginger and Sesame Dressing is gluten free, dairy free and nightshade free but does include soy.

Gluten free, Dairy free, Soy free and Nightshade free Bragg Products:

- Coconut Aminos: Gluten free, dairy free, soy free and nightshade free. Great sub for soy sauce. I will caution that the first time I tasted it I did not like it at all. If you experience that please give it another try in an actual dish. I learned to like it very quickly and I am sure you will too.
- Nutritional Yeast Seasoning: Great sub for parmesan cheese.
- Bragg Organic Apple Cider Vinaigrette: clean!

www.chex.com

Cereal. I want to take this moment to talk about overly processed foods. Like most breakfast cereals, box mixes, etc. Many find that overly processed foods will cause inflammation and pain even though there are not any trigger ingredients listed. If you have eliminated gluten, dairy, nightshades and soy and feel you are still experiencing symptoms I would suggest you try eliminating overly processed foods. Breakfast cereals, box mixes, frozen dinners with long ingredient lists are usually the culprits. We are not sure but the only thing in common could be the artificial ingredients and preservatives.

Chex offers 8 Gluten Free Cereals. I checked the ingredients list of all 8 varieties and they are all gluten free, dairy free, soy free and nightshade free.

Coconut Secret

www.coconutsecret.com

Clean:

- Coconut Secret Coconut Aminos: Gluten free, dairy free, soy free and nightshade free. Great sub for soy sauce. I will caution that the first time I tasted it I did not like it at all. If you experience that please give it another try in an actual dish. I learned to like it very quickly and I am sure you will too.
- Coconut Vinegar is clean. Per their site, the coconut vinegar does not taste like coconut. It has a more pleasant flavor, more mild taste than that of apple cider vinegar.
- Coconut Secret Grain Free Granola Bars

Not completely clean:

- Coconut Secret Hoisin Sauce: gluten free, dairy free and soy free but it does show a small amount of chili powder (a nightshade).
- Coconut Secret Ginger-Turmeric Sauce: gluten free, dairy free and soy free but it does show a small amount of chili powder which is a nightshade.
- Coconut Secret Gochujang Sauce: gluten free, soy free and dairy free but this has smoked paprika and chili powder. Both are nightshades.
- Coconut Secret Garlic Sauce is gluten free, soy free and dairy free but does have cayenne pepper: a nightshade.
- Coconut Secret Teriyaki Sauce: gluten free, dairy free and soy free but it does incudes cayenne: a nightshade.

– www.daiyafoods.com

Clean Products (gluten free, dairy free, nightshade free and soy free)

- Shreds Classic Blend: gluten free, dairy free, soy free and nightshade free.

Shreds: gluten, dairy and soy free but there is a small amount of potato protein. Only a problem for those with a high sensitivity to nightshades. This includes the following Shreds Varieties:

- Cheddar
- Mozzarella

Shreds with potato protein as well as green jalapeno pepper. Both nightshades:

- Pepperjack Style Shreds

Daiya Slices

The following slices varieties are gluten free, dairy free and soy free but includes potato starch as one of the main ingredients.

- Smoked Gouda Slices
- Mozzarella Style Slices
- American Style Slices
- Cheddar Style Slices
- Swiss Style Slices
- Provolone Style

Daiya Block Cheese alternative is the same. All of the varieties are gluten free, dairy free and soy free but all have a bit of potato protein low on the ingredient lists with the Jalapeno Havarti Style Block also having the nightshade jalapeno's.

Daiya Cream Cheez

- Plain Cream Cheez: gluten free, dairy free and soy free but a hint of potato protein.
- Strawberry Cream Cheez: gluten free, dairy free and soy free but a hint of potato protein.
- Chive & Onion Cream Cheez: gluten free, dairy free and soy free but a hint of potato protein.
- Garden Vegetable: While this is gluten free, dairy free and soy free is lists red bell peppers and green bell peppers pretty high on the ingredients list and it also has potato protein. All three are nightshades.

Daiya Frozen Pizza

- Italian Herb & Cheeze Style: Gluten free, dairy free and soy free. Nightshade ingredients: potato starch, potato protein, and tomatoes.

All pizza varieties are gluten and dairy free but include nightshades. Potato in the crust and peppers and tomatoes in the sauce and toppings.

Cheezecake

The cheesecake is gluten and dairy free as well as soy free but does includes nightshades: potato starch is in the filling as well as the crust.

Daiya Cheezy Mac

Clean:
- Deluxe Cheezy Mac Cheddar Style
- Deluxe Cheezy Mac Alfredo Style

Not Clean:

- Deluxe Cheezy Mac White Cheddar Style Veggie: This is gluten, dairy and soy free but it has nightshades: red bell pepper.
- Deluxe Cheezy Mac Meatless Bac'n & Cheddar Style is gluten, dairy and soy free but list a minute amount of paprika near the end of the ingredient list.

- Deluxe Cheezy Mac Four Cheeze Style With Herbs is gluten, dairy and soy free and may be nightshade free. One of the ingredients listed is 'spices'. We don't know what 'spices' actually means and could include some nightshades.

Coconut Yogurt Alternatives:

The yogurt alternatives are gluten, dairy and soy free but list potato starch pretty high up on the ingredients list.

All of the Daiya Dairy Free Dressings have potato starch but are otherwise gluten, dairy and soy free.

Daiya Dairy Free Deluxe Cheeze Sauce Alfredo and Cheddar Style:
- This sauce is Gluten free, dairy free, soy free and nightshade free!
- But the Zesty Cheddar Style Sauce has several nightshades. It is otherwise also gluten, dairy and soy free.

Daiya Frozen Dessert Bars

Gluten free, dairy free, soy free and nightshade free:
- Chocolate Fudge Crunch
- Classic Vanilla Bean
- Salted Caramel Swirl
- Espresso Coffee

Daiya Frozen Burritos

Gluten Free, Dairy Free, Soy Free but not nightshade free:
- Homestyle Breakfast Burrito
- Fiesta Breakfast Burrito
- Santa Fe Burrito
- Santiago Burrito
- Tex-Mex Burrito
- Tuscan Burrito

www.halotop.com

- o Dairy free, gluten free, soy free and nightshade free varieties:
- Birthday Cake
- Candy Bar
- Chocolate
- Chocolate Almond Crunch
- Peanut Butter Cup
- Sea Salt Caramel

- o Dairy Free, Soy Free and Nightshade Free but the following varieties has wheat flour, a gluten, pretty high on the ingredients list:
- Chocolate Chip Cookie Dough

Krusteaz

- www.krusteaz.com

Gluten free, Dairy Free, Soy free and nightshade free Krusteaz products:

Gluten free, dairy free and nightshade free but includes soybean oil pretty high on the ingredients list plus the box has a disclaimer that it 'may contain milk':

- Gluten Free Cinnamon Crumb Cake
- Gluten Free Chocolate Chip Cookie
- Gluten Free Yellow Cake
- Gluten Free Chocolate Cake Mix
- Gluten Free Double Chocolate Brownie

Gluten Free, Soy Free and nightshade free but DOES contain milk; dairy:

- Gluten Free Confetti Buttermilk Pancake Mix

Gluten free and nightshade free but DOES contain dairy and soy:

- Gluten Free Blueberry Muffin
- Gluten Free Buttermilk Pancake mix
- Gluten Free Honey Cornbread

Udi's

– www.udisglutenfree.com

Clean Products that are gluten free, dairy free, soy free and nightshade free:

- o   Bagel: Cinnamon Raisin
- o   Bagel: Everything Bagel
- o   Bagel: Whole Grain Bagels
- o   Sliced Bread: Hearty Sprouted Grains
- o   Sliced Bread: Hearty 7 Seeds & Grain Bread Loaf
- o   Udi's Gluten Free White Sandwich Bread
- o   Whole Grain Bread
- o   Udi's Gluten Free Thin & Crispy Pizza Crusts (the actual Udi's Frozen Pizza's with topping all have dairy and nightshades.)

Products that are gluten free, soy free and nightshade free but do show dairy in the ingredients list:

- o   Udi's Gluten Free English Muffins White
- o   Sausage Breakfast Sandwich (includes dairy cheese)

Products that are gluten free, soy free, and dairy free but include potato starch or potato flour, a nightshade:

- o   Bread: Cinnamon Raisin Bread
- o   Classic French Dinner Rolls
- o   Hot Dog Buns
- o   Hamburger Buns
- o   Gluten Free Plain Tortillas

Gluten Free and Soy Free but DOES includes Nightshades and Dairy:
Frozen Dinner Entrees:
- o   Chicken Frozen Parmesan and Penne
- o   Chicken Alfredo
- o   Italian Sausage Lasagna
- o   Mac & Cheese
- o   Pesto Tortellini

Udi's bread is generally found in the freezer section of the grocery store.

Milton's

–   www.miltonscraftbakers.com

All of the Gluten Free Milton's Crackers contain nightshades in the form of potato and some with added nightshade spices.

Mission

–   www.missionfoods.com

Mission Gluten Free Tortillas are gluten free but do contain soybean oil and nightshades (potato extract, potato starch). Mission tortillas, and many of the other gluten free tortillas are not made to be eaten right out of the package. But a quick warming on both sides in a hot skillet and they are just like a traditional tortilla.

Mission offers products that are gluten free, dairy free, soy free and nightshade free:
- Yellow Corn Tortillas
- White Corn Tortillas
- Baked Tostadas
- Chicharrones Pork rinds Original only. Not flavored.
- Mission Tortilla chips that are not seasoned or flavored like the Restaurant Style Thin & Crispy

Nut Pods Creamer

–   www.nutpods.com

All of the nut pods Creamer varieties are gluten free, dairy free, soy free and nightshade free.

Ronzoni

–   www.ronzoni.com

This is my preferred gluten free pasta brand, I just wish they would go ahead and put out a gluten free lasagna sheet like Barilla. All of the Ronzoni Pasta shapes are clean: gluten free, dairy free, soy free and nightshade free.

Rudi's

www.rudisbakery.com

- All of the Rudi's Gluten Free sliced breads are gluten free, dairy free and soy free but all contain potato starch and flour; a nightshade.

- Rudi's offers two varieties of tortillas, Plain and Spinach Tortillas, are gluten free, dairy free, soy free and nightshade free.

Schar

– www.schaer.com

All of the Shar Gluten Free breads, rolls and sliced breads are gluten free, dairy free and nightshade free. The breads do all contain soy.

The SCHAR Gluten Free PIZZA CRUST ingredients incudes potato starch, a nightshade as well as a statement on the package that it contains Soy.

Silk

www.silk.com

- All of the Silk brand Almond, Cashew and Coconut milks are okay. Avoid the Soymilk as it contains Soy.
- Silk brand makes two Latte varieties and both are clean: gluten free, dairy free, soy free and nightshade free.
- Almond & Oat Latte Mocha and the Espresso flavors. Clean.
- Silk Almond Creamer: all Almond Milk flavors are clean.

Silk also has a Dairy Free Heavy Whipping Cream Alternative and a Half & Half which is clean: gluten free, dairy free, soy free and nightshade free.

Silk has a Soymilk Yogurt alternative, but if you are avoiding soy look for the Almondmilk Yogurt Alterative: They are gluten, dairy, soy and nightshade free.

****

Be sure to go to the Amazon Product page and leave a review! And be sure to check all of my other books. I offer a comprehensive Gluten and Dairy Free Grocery List and a Comprehensive Grocery List that is Gluten Free, Dairy Free, Soy Free and Nightshade Free. Both lists includes brand named package foods from every aisle of the grocery store.

www.amazon.com/author/paulachenderson

www.ingramcontent.com/pod-product-compliance
Lightning Source LLC
Chambersburg PA
CBHW050707250726
48662CB00002B/890